Table of Contents

About the Author

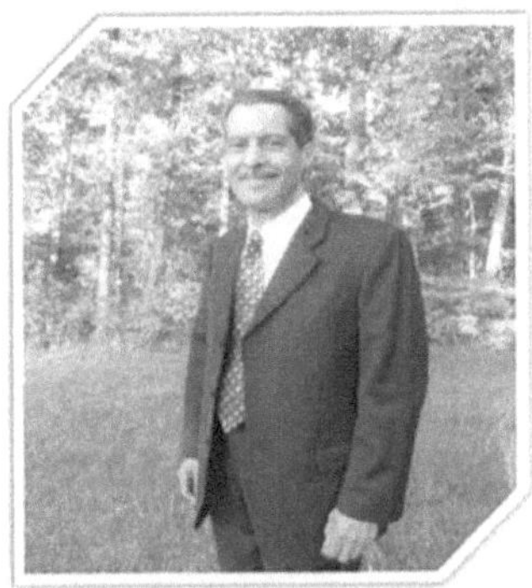 **My name is Jorge Lugo.** I'm an Electrical Engineer (retired). That is how I made my living while I spent decades (since 1964) studying and testing all the diet and health plans covered in popular books and other health and wellness literature. During this time, I developed a health system that increases energy levels while reversing the aging process and its related illnesses. I continue to study the effects of taking extra nutrients and varying my diet for the purpose of optimizing health and physical performance.

I provide health information and solutions that leverage one's metabolism and higher-level metabolic processes to maximize body efficiency. The benefits received from following the suggested healthy lifestyle choices (HLC) that I have identified as being significant in improving health and wellness, will slow the aging process by reversing the aging indicators (hair loss, aging skin, waning libido, arthritis, failing eyesight, muscular atrophy and more).

The aging indicator that provides the basic healthy lifestyle choices and improves your health profile is hair growth.

Learning how to grow and maintain a full head of hair and putting those principles into practice is the first step to better health and slowing the aging process.

About This Book

The purpose of this book is to discuss the theory of how and why hair loss, and the growth and maintenance of a full hairline, is determined by your lifestyle.   It is my view that heredity determines how you grow or lose hair.   However, whether you grow or lose hair is a lifestyle issue.   Unlike other publications on the subject that explain the medical theories of why you lose hair and the different forms of male pattern baldness aimed at helping you more readily accept your plight, I take a different approach.   This book is intended to help you reverse or prevent hair loss and grow and maintain a full head of hair.

I discuss my own trial and error testing that has proven to work for me with the re-growth of my own hair.   Also presented are the results of interviews that I have conducted with men over 50 years of age and one woman in her mid-40s that have full hairlines.   A connection is made between my own hair growth experiences and the information I received from the interviewees to highlight the common lifestyle activity we share. From the evidence presented, I have determined that common lifestyle activity to be exercise.

Also discussed are the negative effects of stress and what it does to our bodies.   Stress adds the dynamic that can undermine our health and ability to grow hair.   Most of you are aware that we need some stress to get us going and keep us motivated throughout the day.   However, you may not be as aware of how low levels of chronic stress can shorten your life, and in the process, reduce the number of hairs on the top of your head.   I will show you how to mitigate stress' damaging effects with recommended levels of activity, diet, and supplementation.

This book also provides a plan to assist you with setting goals for healthy hair growth and how to reach those goals.   The information provided in my plan relating to diet and supplementation coupled with the Metabolic Equivalent (MET) Chart, to assist you with monitoring your level of activity, will insure your success.   When you put the principles covered in this book to work for you, you will stop abnormal hair loss and begin to re-grow and maintain the hairline of your youth.

Introduction

About 38 million people in the United States are experiencing baldness issues.   Most of those people are men but includes a small number of women.   However, virtually all men and women experience thinning of the hair on their heads with age.

The hairline can take years to show the effects of a less than best lifestyle.   It can indicate just how active or inactive an individual has been.   It can also provide valuable information about the stress level and dietary practices of an individual. Throughout the years that I spent learning the causes of hair loss and how to reverse their negative effects, I have identified

other health-aging indicators that are positively affected by an active, healthy lifestyle.   The other health-aging indicators are: Hair color (graying), joint health (arthritis), libido, eye sight strength (macular degeneration), and energy level.   However, the solution to hair growth issues provides the baseline from which to build a healthy lifestyle program that produces positive results with all the health-aging indicators.

My First Hair Loss Story

My interest in hair growth began early in my life.   In 1964 at the age of 16, my barber said to me as he cut my hair, that my hair was thinning.   He also added that I would be bald by the age of 20.   He was referring to the hairline at my forehead.   He really got my attention.

I thought about what the barber told me.   I also thought about my parents and the comments they made from time to time about hair loss.   My parents were intelligent people with great powers of observation.   My parents often said that people can lose hair and have their hair go gray due to being overwhelmed by stress.   I had also heard doctors on the radio say that walking can help to lower the stress in one's life.   I put the two thoughts together and decided to try walking to lower the stress that I assumed was causing my hair to thin.

I walked everywhere.   I lived in Brooklyn, New York at the time and was too young to drive a car, so I had to walk wherever I needed to go.   I took every opportunity to walk.   I would walk to

speak to a friend half a mile away instead of calling by phone. Consequently, at my follow-on visits to my barber every month, I heard no more about thinning hair.   The walking program was working for me. However, that was not the end of the story.   I learned over the following years that there are other factors involved in the process that also need to be considered and managed, though one's level of activity is a key factor.

The Interviews

I decided to conduct interviews with men who have full heads of hair and that were old enough to make their full hairlines stand out.   Interviewing and studying men with full heads of hair made more sense to me than interviewing and studying balding men. I was not interested in learning the reasons why men become bald.   Rather, I was interested in learning why some men grow and maintain full heads of hair.

I concentrated my efforts in identifying those lifestyle habits that would make it possible for me to continue growing a strong, full head of hair.   Just like with my first episode with hair loss at the age of 16, I wanted to have a plan in place to prevent future episodes of hair loss.

In the early 1990s, I interviewed several of my colleagues at my office building in Washington, DC.   The interviews were informal.   After all, I was at the office to work.   I targeted each of the individuals because they each had a great hairline.   I would catch each of them at lunch or on their way out of the building to a meeting, etc.   My questions were about the activities they enjoyed, what they ate, and at what times they did these things throughout the day.   I also asked them about the stress level in their lives.

It was interesting to me that when it came to what they ate, I could not find any one thing or things that I could point to that account for their great hairlines.   I also could not identify any significant stress or stressful events in their lives.   They appeared to have good eating habits and well-balanced lives with no heavy emotional issues.   Their level of activity, however, was a different matter.

Most of the interviewees were men because men historically have a greater tendency than women to lose their hair.   This fact is due to men having more of the hormone testosterone than women.   However, women may not be as likely to experience hair loss but do remain at risk depending upon their lifestyle.   None of us are immune from experiencing the stress that abounds in life.   Consequently, I focused my attention on men.   However, my expectation was that the factors that positively affect the growth of hair on men are the same hair growth factors that will make it easier for women to grow and maintain fuller, thicker heads of hair.

Ozzie E, Dave H, and Jay J

Ozzie and Dave walked every evening for about an hour.   Jay did not.   According to the responses I received from Jay, it appeared that it did not matter at what time of the day I walked because he walked around noon time every day.   I decided to walk during my lunch break for about an hour and it did not work for me.

How did I know it wasn't working for me?   Since my mid-30s my hair loss has been gradual.   At that time, my high level of activity during my 20s came to a sudden halt when I injured myself lifting heavy furniture in late 1978.   That event triggered the beginning of my hair loss.   I began noticing the hair loss about 5 years after I injured myself.   I slowly worked at getting back to the level of activity I maintained prior to late 1978.   However, my injury made that impossible.   Instead, I was half as active as I was prior to 1978.   The good news was that my new level of activity was enough to slow down the rate at which I was losing hair to a gradual pace.   Consequently, I have been able to visually monitor the progress of my hairline on a weekly basis.

The Jay J Story

Jay was one of the individuals that I interviewed who appeared to not fit the mold.   That is, Jay did not walk during the evenings like the first two men that I interviewed.   Jay walked during his lunch break around noon time.   Given that Jay was walking for exercise and he did have a full hairline, my first thought was that perhaps the time of the day that one exercises does not matter.

I tested the premise.   Every day, I walked around lunchtime for about an hour.   I would schedule my work-day so I would discuss business matters with colleagues in other buildings near my office before or after noon time.

This was an enjoyable experience.   It was a great way of getting re-energized and being more productive work-wise in the afternoon.   Unfortunately, it did nothing to help me increase the thickness of my hairline.   I did everything I could to make it work.   I changed my lunchtime routine by eating before I began my walk.   I tried eating during my walk by beginning my walk then eating lunch, then completing my walk.   If you are sensing some frustration on my part, it is because it was frustrating.   I decided to speak with Jay again when he had some time to let him know that the noontime walks were not working for me.   I would also ask Jay if there is something unique about his diet or other lifestyle issue that he would like to share with me.

I caught up with Jay and he had some time to talk.   It had been a few months since my first discussion with him.   Jay must have spent some time thinking about our previous discussion because when I began asking him questions, he surprised me with the quickness of his answers.   No sooner I mentioned that I tried walking during noon time and that it didn't work for me, he replied that he also plays basketball during the evenings several times a week.

I was genuinely relieved to hear Jay say this because participating in basketball games is a high aerobic activity.   This revelation reminded me of my karate practices several times a week during the evening some 20 years earlier (1967).

Jay confirmed for me that his level of activity was high enough, particularly at the end of the day, to sustain growing a full hairline.   His level of activity was higher than the level of activity of the other 2 men.   It now became clear to me why I faired so well over the years with growing and maintaining a full head of hair.   It was my high level of activity (karate) during the evenings that paid off in a big way for me.

The information that Jay shared with me was exciting news. However, as I tried to get back into the high aerobic karate practices, I found myself unable to keep up.   I simply had too many responsibilities that left me at the end of the day with insufficient energy to cope with strenuous exercise.   I needed to find an exercise solution with lifestyle changes that fit my daily routine.   I knew this was possible because the men that I interviewed were all growing great heads of hair while expending a minimum amount of energy exercising.

My Exercise Program

My high aerobic exercise routine was the reason behind my thick hairline.   In 1967, I began practicing karate at a dojo.   I was 19 years old.   Let me make this point clear.   I was no Bruce Lee or Chuck Norris.   It was just an interesting activity that ended 2 years later.   At the same time, I was studying Electrical Engineering at the Polytechnic Institute of Brooklyn (today the Polytechnic University) and did not have the energy to keep up with both karate practice and my studies.   I therefore chose to give up karate practice at the dojo.   I did, however, continue the karate exercises because they were a great aerobic workout. Within several years of beginning my karate practice, I was growing hair so thick that I was the envy of those with full hairlines as well as those who were bald.

Unfortunately, I did not know back then all I know today about diet and water intake.   Instead, I relied upon shear will power to keep me going in a perpetual state of dehydration.   As a result, I suffered with bouts of dry skin and low carbohydrate stores that caused physical and mild mental lethargy.   In other words, I was a walking zombie from time to time.   However, I grew and maintained a phenomenal head of hair.   I eventually realized that I had failed to maintain the proper balance between exercise, diet, and hydration.

As I looked back at my early 20s, I saw there is a connection between hair growth and level of activity (exercise). However, the level of activity I maintained during my 20s was unrealistic in terms of the physical and mental energy it cost to maintain. As I matured and took on more responsibilities at home and the office, I could no longer afford to continue the same level of exercise. Like myself, I strongly suspect that most of you are not interested in expending that much energy and time for the sole purpose of growing and maintaining a full head of hair either. To solve that problem, I began a quest to find a solution to growing and maintaining a full head of hair that incorporates achievable exercise routines and lifestyle changes.

The Dave C Story

As far as hairlines go, Dave C's was to die for. He has the hairline of a 12-year-old boy. However, when I asked Dave if he exercised, his response was no. I then asked Dave C if he walks for exercise. Dave's response again was no. He explained to me that he does not exercise at all.

His responses literally left me scurrying back to the drawing board to figure this one out. One possible explanation could have been that Dave C is genetically predisposed to growing and maintaining a full head of hair. That was not likely, since I have determined that hair growth is a direct result of one's lifestyle. However, it could be that Dave C just isn't affected by stress. He could be one of those rare individuals that just doesn't worry about anything and therefore has a perpetually low stress response.

I thought about Dave C from time to time over the following year. I saw Dave C on occasion leaving and entering the office building and I would engage him in small talk hoping he might provide a clue as to why he is growing a phenomenal head of hair without exercising.   Eventually, it occurred to me that hair loss takes time and therefore it was possible that Dave C has engaged in some form of exercise in the past.   I decided to approach Dave C with a new set of questions.

I approached Dave C again about a year after I posed my first questions to him.   This time the focus of my questions was centered on his past exercise activities.   In addition, I had other questions to ask him about his diet.   I first asked Dave C if he has ever engaged in any form of exercise and he responded yes. Dave explained to me that he was doing resistance training workouts.   His resistance training workouts were several hours a day five to six days a week.   He also added that he did resistance training for about 20 years.

As I spoke with Dave, I realized that my informal interviews were not long enough.   On an informal basis, I did not have enough time to ask enough of the right questions to get the complete health history of the interviewees.   Dave C was a perfect example of this.   Fortunately, I kept track of the questions and responses over the year it took for me to get the complete picture of Dave C's lifestyle activities.

The last question I asked Dave was, when did he stop his weight training.   He said he did so 2 years before.   This means that when I first approached Dave C, he had stopped exercising a year before. Now it all made sense. Enough time had not passed with Dave C being inactive for him to experience hair thinning. I advised Dave that if he continues to be inactive, he will notice hair beginning to fall out at a higher rate than normal and will see areas of thinning hair about 5 to 7 years from the time he stopped exercising.

The Hair Growth Cycle

An explanation of the hair growth cycle provides an understanding of the process not only of hair growth but also of hair loss and the re-growth of lost hair. As the dynamics of the hair growth process are presented, your ability to visualize the time element involved will help you cope with the process of re-growing a full head of hair. The good news is that by following my Plan, you can reduce the amount of time it takes to turn hair loss into the re-growth of a full hair line. Therefore, understanding the hair growth process and accepting the fact that my Plan will help you re-grow hair quickly, will make following the Plan easier.

Hair growth occurs in phases. The process is documented in books. There are three phases of hair growth. They are the growing phase, the shrinking phase, and the resting phase. The growth phase lasts from 4 to 6 years. During the growth phase, the new hair will push out the old hair if it has not fallen out already. The new hair will grow to its full thickness and length. About 85 – 90 percent of all the hair on your head are in the growing phase at any moment in time.

The shrinking phase happens next.   During the shrinking phase, the hair stops growing and the hair follicle starts shrinking.   The hair follicle and hair bulb disintegrate, and the hair just sits in the scalp with no support structure to help keep it there.   If the hair doesn't fall out during the 2 to 3 week period of time that the shrinking phase lasts, then the new hair will push out the old hair when the growth cycle begins anew.   The percentage of hair in this phase is about 3 to 4 percent.

The resting phase begins after the hair follicle stops shrinking. During this phase is when most old hair is shed.   The shedding of old hair occurs at a rate of 50 – 100 hairs a day.   About 13 percent of all the hair on your head are in the resting phase at any given time.   The resting phase normally lasts 5 – 6 weeks.

The periods of time noted above for the hair growth phases are for normal hair growth.   The periods of time and hair dynamics change when the body experiences chronic stress including chronic low levels of stress.   As the hair follicle is starved of blood flow and nutrients due to a higher stress response, the growth phase gets shorter with the hair length growing shorter and the diameter of the hair shaft growing smaller with every full growth cycle.   Reduce the stress response and more blood flow with vital nutrients for healthy hair growth reach the hair follicle. Consequently, as more blood and nutrients reach the hair follicle, the hair growth cycle begins to get longer, and the hair shaft grows towards its full length and thickness.

As we practice less than best diet regimens and exercise less frequently, we experience varying degrees of hair loss at a random pace.   However, by understanding the basic principles of hair growth, and applying the principles consistently, the rate of re-growth of hair is maximized.   In other words, the hair that took 10 years to lose can be regained in 2-3 years.

I provide this caveat to keep you from misunderstandings as to what my hair growth program can help you accomplish.   When you begin following my program, you will notice new hair growth within 30 days.   Some of the hair growth, particularly at the crown of the head and the frontal part of the head may fall out prematurely.   These are the areas of the head that are affected more by stress and therefore will take the longest to return to normal hair growth.

This has been my experience with the re-growth of my own hair. Reversing general thinning has been relatively easy for me as I follow my Plan.   However, getting the hair at the crown area and temples of my head to re-grow has proven to take more time.

The Steve M Story

Steve was a relatively young man.   When I first spoke with Steve about my hair growth Plan, he was 29 years old.   Steve had lost a considerable amount of hair on the top and front of his head. Steve shared with me that he was not happy with his hair loss.

Steve was so unhappy with his hair loss that he had a hair transplant.

The transplant was comprised of a series of hair plugs taken from the back of his head and transplanted in a semi-circular line near his original hairline at his forehead.   His plan was to have several follow-on visits to his surgeon to transplant additional hair plugs behind the transplants he showed me.   I remember Steve said he paid $2,500.00 for his transplant (early 1990s).

I shared with Steve what I was learning about hair and the re-growth of hair.   I told Steve about the interviews I conducted with men over 50 years of age, and my own experimentation with diet and supplementation to obtain a healthy synergy that would make growing hair easier even when subjected to stressful situations.   Steve mentioned that he noticed my hairline receding some around my temples and that over time he noticed my hair had grown back.   For this reason, Steve embraced my Plan and decided to put my plan into action.

At that point, I had a formidable wealth of hands-on knowledge about hair growth and compelling evidence that when applied works.   I provided Steve with instructions on the lifestyle changes necessary for the re-growth of his hair.   I asked Steve to walk every evening because that is what the first three men over 50 with full heads of hair that I interviewed were doing.   I also asked Steve to switch to a diet that is lower in concentrated protein (meat, fish or chicken) and to eat meals comprised mainly of carbohydrates at dinner time.

Steve came by to visit several weeks after he began following my plan. As we spoke, he pulled his hair back at his forehead and showed me his hair re-growing in front of the hair plugs he had transplanted. I was excited to say the least. Now I had proof that my observations and theories worked not only on me but on others also. I was encouraged to continue experimenting to find easier ways to apply my working theories while maximizing the results that could be achieved.

Steve stopped following my plan because it was restrictive. I did not know enough then to be able to offer diet choices to Steve. I decided then that I needed to focus more time and energy on developing flexible eating guidelines that provide the users of my plan with a variety of food choices.

The Emma H Story

There are many people that I spoke with about their lifestyle activities because of their great hairlines. All those people that I informally interviewed were men except for one. Her name is Emma. My meeting and ultimate interview with Emma was a chance meeting in mid-2003. I spoke with Emma and her husband at their house in Williamsburg, Virginia.

My wife and I decided upon a house plan for our retirement home. Emma and her husband built and lived in the same style house. My wife contacted Emma and her husband, and we were invited to visit them and walk through their house. I was very pleased with the thought of visiting and seeing what our future house would look like.

Upon our arrival, it was Emma's husband that I met first. He was busy working on the outside of the house. The first thing that I noticed about Emma's husband was his strong, thick hairline. However, by this time I had enough interviews with males that support my findings on the relationship between level of activity and hair growth. I didn't need to address the subject of hairlines with Emma's husband – particularly since I barely knew him. However, all that changed when I met Emma. Like her husband, she also had a strong, thick hairline.

I had not seen a couple where both were growing thick hairlines. At this point, my curiosity was peaked. This may be a situation where a common diet practice could be at work. If so, by identifying that common diet practice would make the Plan more powerful. I decided then to make a gutsy move and steer the conversation with Emma and her husband in the direction of health and hair growth.

I refer to my decision as gutsy because my wife had asked me - in a firm tone of voice - not to bring up the subject of health with Emma and her husband. We were there to walk through the house and show our gratitude by being as gracious as possible to them.

Emma's husband was busy working on the house, so it was Emma that completed the walk through with us.   During the walk through, I was thinking about how I could introduce the subject of health into the conversation without upsetting my wife.   Then, as we were ready to bid our farewells, my wife stepped outside to ask Emma's husband a few questions.   I took that opportunity to let Emma know how healthy she and her husband looked.   I shared with her that my hobby turned passion is health and wellness.   I asked her about their diet and supplementation practices.   I also asked what type of exercise they engage in.

Emma was genuinely interested in the conversation on health. This encouraged me to quickly move on to talking about Emma and her husband's hairlines before my wife returned.   Emma had no diet or supplementation information to share with me that stands out as the reason for their great hairlines.   She did, however, share with me that she and her husband walk together to Colonial Williamsburg and back virtually every evening. Depending on how far they walk, it takes them about 40 minutes to an hour.

I should have ended the conversation then, before my wife returned.   Instead, I continued by sharing with Emma the discussions I had with the men I interviewed to highlight how important her and her husband's walks are for their obvious good health and hairlines.   Consequently, towards the end of the conversation, my wife did walk back into the house.   I quickly wrapped up the discussion and apologized to Emma for getting overly involved in a conversation on health.   We thanked Emma and her husband for their kindness and left.   My wife was not happy that I ignored her wishes.

The Stress Response and Hair Growth

It's important to understand the body's stress response, and why I relate all the health planning and its associated activities to it.   The stress response is pivotal in relation to the external stresses we experience every day.   Although we have little control over the daily stress we are exposed to in our lives, we do have control over our stress response to those external stimuli.   In addition, we do have control over the lifestyle choices we make that can affect our stress response.

The stress response is what physically occurs within the body when it is subjected to a stressful situation.   The stress response can be viewed as the agitation the body experiences due to stress.   The stress response rises and falls in direct proportion to the rise and fall of insulin level in our bodies caused by the release of the stress hormone Cortisol.   In simpler terms, the stress response of the body follows the up and down swings of insulin in the body.   The higher the insulin level, the higher the stress response and vice versa.

The scientific research has established that when your insulin levels rise, you are under physical stress.   There is a physical connection and not just a psychosomatic response.   The reaction by the body is the "fight-flight" response.   The "fight-flight" response also causes the blood vessels on the surface of the skin to constrict thereby reducing blood flow to the extremities and diverts that blood flow to the vital organs – a key to survival in a fight scenario.   Physically, you have gone into high gear.   Your body depletes its vitamins, minerals and water stores more quickly.   Combine that with less blood circulating at the top of your head and you experience hair loss.

Diet and Hair Growth

Analyzing Steve's story, the results that he achieved confirmed that exercise and diet do affect the hair growth process. Exercise can make a difference in whether we grow or lose hair. Steve confirmed that one's diet can determine how much or how little exercise we need to engage in for strong hair growth. When Steve switched to a vegetarian diet, his meals were digested more easily.   His stress response was lowered to the point that a low level of activity in the evening was enough to effect hair growth.   Steve combined a more vegetarian diet with a slightly higher level of activity (walking) and produced amazing results.   He began to re-grow his hair in front of the transplanted hair plugs.

During my trial and error testing of various diets and exercise routines between the years 1990 to the present, I have reached

the conclusion that exercise can overcome a less than best diet.
In other words, you can exercise strenuously enough to
overcome the stresses that modern day society and poor diet
practices may cause.   However, the synergy achieved between
a well-managed diet and exercise program can make the
process of growing and maintaining a full head of hair easier to
achieve as well as beneficial to your health.

My preferred methodology to finding a solution to hair loss has
been, and remains today, those practices that promote a healthy
lifestyle.   The practices that I have incorporated into my Plan for
hair growth follow the health principles proven to work over time.
Exercise and a properly balanced diet supported by adequate
supplementation are at the heart of my Plan.   These are the
same practices that provide me with improved health and
promotes the growth of my full hairline.

Supplementation and Hair Growth

Scientific research tells us the nutrients that we receive from the
foods we eat are necessary to provide our bodies with energy
and the building blocks for repair and growth.   The research
also supports the theory that additional amounts of some
vitamins and minerals can prevent the damaging effects of free
radicals caused by poor diet, environmental pollution, and

stress.   These are not new theories that require decades of testing for verification.   The theories were researched and published in the 1950s through 1970s, when they first appeared in scientific journals and popular magazines.

The first theory that I read on health was a magazine article titled, The Free Radical Theory of Aging.   I remember that being around 1964.   It was explained in layman's terms that there are free radicals produced when normal cells split into two.   The free radicals are missing an electron and will seek and attach themselves to healthy cells making them unstable.   This all sounds very orderly and good.   Unfortunately, when free radicals attach to healthy cells, it alters the cells.   The altered cells are damaged and produce more free radicals when they split into two.   The net effect on the body is degeneration and aging, because we lose more cells than are generated.

The article went on to explain how vitamins C and E and the mineral Selenium if present in adequate amounts neutralize the free radicals by providing the electrons they need.   The net effect of this antioxidant vitamin and mineral rich scenario is regeneration of the body.   It reverses aging because there are more cells produced than cells lost.

Over the years that followed to this present day, I have not read an article or publication that contradicts the free radical theory of aging. What I have read are articles in support of the theory that have expanded the list of vitamins and minerals that play a role in the process.

As I continue to read books and publications on health, I have concluded that reversing aging is not dependent solely on the neutralization of free radicals in the body. To achieve regeneration of cells to the point where you will notice higher energy levels, more youthful looking skin, and hair re-growth also requires improving the systems that deliver and process the nutrients. This is where higher levels of activity and properly balanced diet enter the picture. However, without a comprehensive supplementation program working for you, the results you can achieve in reversing the health-aging indicators including hair growth may be limited.

Vitamins and minerals in adequate amounts promote the efficiency of the body. They provide for a high state of readiness in which the body can accomplish regeneration unimpeded. A case in point is the mineral Zinc. Zinc is important for the health of the prostate in men. Zinc is found in high concentrations in the prostate. A deficiency in Zinc can also cause hair loss. Can it be that part of the hair loss problem in men is due to inadequate levels of Zinc required for hair growth which may be due to the prostate competing for available stores of Zinc? I believe so and will discuss the relationship of Zinc to hair growth as well as other diet and nutrition topics in more depth in a future publication.   Meanwhile, suffice it to say that getting adequate amounts of the essential and non-essential nutrients required by the body for good health is a good idea if you want to grow and maintain a full head of hair more easily.

My Plan provides a list of nutrients that have worked for me in successfully growing and maintaining a strong hairline.   The nutrients have also been instrumental in providing me with additional health benefits that have helped me maintain a healthier lifestyle free from the common cold and other illnesses.

By now, some of you may be wondering what supplements I use. My supplements of choice are produced by Shaklee Corporation. Their products provide me with consistent, high quality nutrition that is backed by independent scientific research.   I also use nutrition products purchased from the local pharmacy.

MET Chart

A copy of the MET Chart is a free download via my Smartphone and Tablet APP, healthylc.   The MET is a representation of the "Metabolic Equivalent".   It is the standardized scientific measure of an activity's caloric burn rate in calories per kilogram per hour. Its usefulness to you is the ability to determine how one activity fairs against other activities in terms of energy usage. For example: Sleeping has a MET of 0.9 while standing quietly is 1.2 and sitting quietly is 1.0. Walking at 2 miles per hour is represented by a MET of 2.0 while biking at less than 10 mph is 4.0. What this means is when you are walking you are burning twice as many calories as when sitting quietly. Biking requires 4 times more energy when compared to sitting quietly but only twice as much when compared to walking. The MET can help you choose the exercises that are best for you to meet your fitness goals. It also helps you view other equivalent exercises (same MET number) as a substitute exercise/daily activity allowing for changes to your routine.

The ability to substitute equivalent energy exercises is an important feature of the MET Chart. It is easy for people to lose their interest in their exercise program because of boredom. By knowing the MET number for different activities, you can add daily routines such as walking during the day at work, vacuuming the house when at home, or hand washing/waxing the car to increase the number of calories you burn and thereby avoid boredom. The increase in rate of calories burned by adding higher levels of activity such as vacuuming also count towards meeting your exercise goals.

Putting It All Together

Successfully growing a full head of hair is about overcoming the stresses that life throws your way.   I overcome those stresses through an exercise program supported by a balanced diet and supplementation choices that help me to maintain a low stress response.   It is the achievement of a low stress response that moves the body from an unhealthy fight-flight response state to a relaxed healthy state.   When the body is relaxed, it requires fewer nutrients and less water, thus maintaining proper hydration and higher stores of the nutrients that can be utilized for the growth of hair.

The process of growing hair involves understanding the lifestyle activity that the interviewees mentioned earlier have in common. That activity is exercise.   In the case of the first 3 interviewees, the exercise is walking.   Therefore, a good starting point in the process is walking every evening for about an hour.   The starting point can be any activity that has a MET of around 3.5. This starting point in the process is the logical first step since Ozzie and Dave H both walked most evenings for about one hour.   The third interviewee, Jay, walked for about an hour during his lunch break virtually every day, and supplemented that activity with basketball sessions in the evenings.   They are all doing just fine maintaining full hairlines.

However, these examples of higher levels of activity don't tell the whole story.   I have tested the theory that walking alone is all that is needed to grow and maintain a full hairline, and it did not work for me all the time.   The conclusion I reached is, there are other factors involved in the process that need to be identified.

As I continued to monitor and test different exercise routines over the years, I realized there are only 2 other variables that I can control that make a difference in whether I was growing hair or losing hair.   The two variables are diet and supplementation. My second realization was the importance of timing in everything that I was doing.   Whether it was the type of exercise I was engaged in, what I was eating, or the supplements I was taking, the time of the day that I engaged in the activities determined whether I was growing or losing hair.

A properly balanced diet with the proper portions timed to take advantage of your body's metabolism will maintain a low stress response and therefore promote the growth of hair.   The same principle applies to exercise.   It is preferable to engage in resistance training when your metabolism is high.   Engaging in resistance type exercises when your metabolism is low raises your stress response.   Raising your stress response means you need to engage in low aerobic activities such as walking, vacuuming, washing the car, or any combination of these activities for longer than an hour to bring your stress response back down into the healthy range.

Of the two variables that affect the hair growth process, I have eliminated supplementation.   I rely on high quality supplements to provide me with the nutrition that my body requires.   The products that I use every day provide, at a minimum, the essential vitamins and minerals that my body needs.   In addition, the supplementation program that I developed goes beyond providing just the basics.   I take additional vitamins, food supplements, and herbs to lower the inflammation and risk of disease my body is exposed to which also lowers my stress response.   This proactive supplementation program maximizes body efficiency and consistently provides for the ability to grow and maintain a strong hairline.

With supplementation eliminated as a hair growth variable, diet is the one other variable that needs to be managed.   As with Steve, he combined his walking routine with a strict vegetarian diet in order to effect hair growth.   It worked so well that he began re-growing hair in front of his transplanted plugs.   Steve would not have accomplished this amazing feat, if he had not included the dietary changes that I recommended along with his increasing his level of activity by walking every evening.   In fact, I intentionally asked Steve to change his diet in addition to walking, because I had discovered that a vegetarian diet is more easily digested and can make a difference with the process of hair growth.

Before running off to begin a vegetarian diet for the purpose of growing hair more easily, remember that Steve discontinued his vegetarian diet due to boredom.   He wasn't raised a vegetarian, so he lacked the knowledge and experience needed to help him make food choices that he liked.   If you believe you can successfully manage adding more vegetarian foods to your diet, then you should make the change.   It is easier to grow a full head of hair on a vegetarian fair.   However, it isn't necessary to follow a vegetarian diet to grow hair.   You can exercise harder and longer to compensate for the less than best diet choices you make.

To illustrate this point: Dave was resistance training 5 to 6 days a week with each session several hours long.   I maintain that Dave C's metabolism was high enough that it would have been difficult for him to reverse its positive effects due to poor diet practices.   Dave C's exercises had a MET of at least 5.   Dave's rate of calories burned during the twenty years he was active doing resistance training is impressive.   He was able to grow and maintain the hairline of a boy of 12 regardless of his dietary practices.   The shear bulk of food he needed to fuel his level of activity every day provided the nutrients his body needed for the growth of hair.

Dave C's concentrated efforts on resistance training lowered his stress response into the healthy range and kept it there.   I find that working out several hours a day, 5 to 6 days a week to be remarkable.   As I stated earlier, I used to work out for 90 minutes several times a week.   Eventually, I stopped the high intensity (aerobic) work outs because of an injury that I sustained in late 1978.   As I got older, I also found that I did not have the time or energy to return to exercising at such a high intensity.   My character and mental state of being make it unlikely that I would be able to accomplish what Dave C has done.   When I think that he continued his high level of activity for twenty years, I am astounded.

Dave C is truly unique in this regard.   He had the fortitude and tenacity to engage in heavy, long term exercise that afforded him the hairline of a child of 12.   However, this is an impractical expectation for most of us to achieve.   I suspect that most of you have very busy lifestyles that leave little time to devote to long exercise sessions solely for the purpose of growing and maintaining a full head of hair.

Fortunately, I spent years – and continue to do so - experimenting with different exercise, diet, and supplementation routines to efficiently achieve the growth and maintenance of a full head of hair with the least amount of effort.   My Plan in combination with the MET Chart can help you meet this time and energy-on-a-budget exercise program.   It is also beneficial to combine the synergy of exercise, diet, and supplementation to manage the re-growth of hair because it provides for a healthier lifestyle that can reverse all the health-aging indicators.

My Plan leverages the timing of the things that we do to take full advantage of the metabolic cycles of the body.   Many of the publications I have read on metabolism point to the broad application of a general theory or principle in a specific area of health.   Unfortunately, the body has numerous functions and processes at work at any given time.   Applying a theory or principle too broadly without consideration given to timing does not work well.   For example, the theory that maintaining a 1:1 carbohydrate-protein ratio (Zone Diet) is healthy and therefore should be applied to every meal does not take advantage of other metabolic processes.   The application of this theory will not help you grow muscle efficiently.   Applying the 1:1 carbohydrate-protein ratio to every meal can eventually cause muscle loss that may lead to loss of bone mass and elevated blood pressure.

The missing part of the logic behind the 1:1 carbohydrate-protein ratio theory is it does not account for the recovery and growth of muscle.   Muscle growth is maximized by consuming a meal that contains a 2.7:1 carbohydrate-protein ratio immediately after a work-out.   The ratio is slightly higher for endurance athletes looking for improved performance as well as muscular recovery.   The ratio for recovery from endurance type activities is closer to 4:1 ratio.   I prefer eating a snack comprised of a 1;1 ratio, and one meal at a ratio of 3:1.   In addition, I eat a light fair of carbohydrates late in the day.   This is what works best for me.

The principle of timing also applies to exercise.   When you exercise becomes just as important as whether you do or don't exercise.   Add to the equation the amount of time spent engaged in a type of exercise, and the amount of time spent exercising determines the best time of the day to engage in that exercise.   For instance, I enjoy my high aerobic exercise and resistance training (high MET) early in the day and low aerobic (low MET) late in the day.   This approach allows my body to recover throughout the day from the high stress activities I engaged in earlier in the day.

The same principle holds true for the diet and supplementation choices you make.   When you make specific choices in the types of foods and portions you eat, knowing the time of the day to eat specific foods and the portions of those foods to eat, provides you with a health advantage.   Likewise, the same principle applies to the vitamins and minerals that you take as supplements.   I eat large meals with proteins during the day and have several snacks instead of dinner.   I take the bulk of my supplements during the middle part of the day when my metabolism is at its highest.   This is the essence of timing.

My Plan and MET Chart incorporate the sum of the knowledge that I have acquired relative to growing and maintaining a full head of hair.   The Plan and MET Chart provides a systematic approach to increasing your body's efficiency, counter the negative effects of stress, and provide you with the ability to grow and maintain the hairline of your youth.

My Hair Growth Plan

NOTE: Before making changes to your diet, exercise or supplementation program, it is recommended that you consult with your health care professional before making any changes.

My Plan focuses on increasing your level of activity. It is higher levels of activity that provide for a lower stress response. In other words, your stress response determines how high your level of activity needs to be. Higher levels of activity that are engaged in on a regular basis provide for the ability to grow and maintain a full head of hair. Therefore, if you are losing hair you need to increase your level of activity.

There are numerous lifestyle issues that affect your stress response. Once again, the first step is exercise. You begin the process with a higher level of activity that aligns with Ozzie and Dave H at the low end of the MET scale and work towards increasing your level of activity to meet that of Dave C at the higher end of the MET. When you begin to see signs of strong hair growth, you have attained the MET number that works for you. By employing this process, you avoid over-exercising.

The MET Chart ranges from 1.5 to 18.0. Although the MET Chart provides very high energy exercises, the time element involved with recovery activities make those exercise scenarios unlikely and not recommended for the average person.

Understanding the relationship between the activities that you enjoy doing and their corresponding MET number is important for starting and maintaining an exercise program.   Through the frequent use of the MET, you can become proficient at associating exercise routines with their MET number.

Determining Your Baseline MET

1. **Obtain a free copy of the MET Chart.**
    a. Download the Smartphone and Tablet APP, healthylc. It's a free download from the APP Store or Google Play.
    b. In the APP, lower right corner, Click "More"
    c. Click "Downloads"
    d. Click "MET Chart"
    e. Click "Download Now"

2. **Already growing a full head of hair:**
    a. Pick the daily activities you engage in every day to determine your baseline MET number.   Include activities you engage in at the gym, around the house and on the job.
    b. Write down the estimated number of minutes that you spend performing the activities you chose.
    c. Continue with those activities.

3. **Losing hair at an abnormal rate:**
    a. Pick the activities that you engage in at the gym, around the house and on the job.
    b. Write down the number of minutes that you spend performing the activities you chose.
    c. Engage in an activity that has a MET number of 3.5 or higher for a minimum of 40 minutes per day, 3 times a week.   Work your way up to 40 minutes to avoid injury.   Ex: Walking with purpose (3.0mph) is a good start.
    d. If new hair growth does not begin to show within 2 weeks, then increase your exercise time or begin an exercise with a higher MET number.
    e. Repeat Steps a through d.

Check your hairline and reevaluate your level of activity periodically.   Checking your hairline and corresponding MET will provide you with a visual indication and representative number that will assist you with growing and maintaining a strong and full hairline.

There will be no guesswork involved in deciding what steps to take to turn around hair loss resulting from the stressful changes that can occur in your life at any age.   When life issues become tougher to handle, causing an increase in your stress response and corresponding hair loss, you increase your level of activity to correspond with the required higher MET number.

When everything is going your way and you are feeling stress free, then lowering your level of activity to a lower MET number may be the appropriate action.

My Supplementation Program

Before beginning a program that involves increasing your level of activity, there are other factors to be considered.   The first is maintaining your body operating at high efficiency.   The second is following dietary guidelines that help you maintain a low stress response.

For your body to operate in a highly efficient state, it needs to receive the basic level of nutrition that allows for the multitude of metabolic processes required by the body to occur.   The body also needs additional nutrients to counter the pollutants, bacteria, and viruses that can interfere with the metabolic processes required for a healthy body and ultimately the growth of a full hairline.

These nutrients come in the form of vitamins and minerals (micronutrients) and we receive them in the foods that we eat.

However, the scientific research questions the amounts of micronutrients found in our food.   Due to transit times and exposure to heat and light, the micronutrient content of the foods we eat is low at best.   Therefore, supplementation becomes the viable option.

Food supplementation is nothing new.   In 1795, English sailors on the high seas had their diets supplemented with lemons (eventually limes and lime juice was added) to prevent scurvy which is caused by a lack of vitamin C.   English sailors suffered with bouts of scurvy for about 300 years until Dr. James Lind discovered the connection between lemons and limes and scurvy in 1747.   Prior to Dr. Lind's discovery, claims were made by casual observers that lemons and limes added to the diet can prevent the disease.   However, no action was taken by the British Navy until after Dr. Lind's death.   Today, the lag time between observed deduction and medical research that establishes a wellness claim and the medical establishment accepting the claim as fact is about 30 years.

An example that highlights this 30-year lag time is Mr. Nathan Pritikin and the best-selling books he wrote on reversing heart disease back in the 1960s and 1970s.   Mr. Pritikin popularized existing research claiming that the lack of exercise, and diets too high in animal protein and lacking in fruits and vegetables are the cause of heart disease.   I recall that doctors responding to Mr. Pritikin's claims were incensed due to his lack of a medical degree.   Mr. Pritikin was an Inventor/Engineer.   However, about thirty years later in the 1990s doctors were asking their

patients to become more active, eat less red meat and dairy and
more vegetables and fruit to lower their risk of heart disease.
Mr. Pritikin began a diet revolution that added years to the lives
of many people with heart disease and kept some from
experiencing heart problems.

Today, we supplement our diets not just with fruits and
vegetables but with vitamins, minerals, and herbs.   The
vitamins and minerals provide the essential and non-essential
vitamins and minerals that our diets may lack.   Herbs, on the
other hand, increase our body's ability to cleanse itself and
resist illness more effectively.

My Plan begins with the following basic nutrition:

   Multivitamin-mineral tablet – 1 per day.

   Vita C chewable, 500mg tablets – 1 to 2 per day.

   B-Complex – 2 to 4 per day.

   Vitamin E, 400 IU – 1 caplet/tablet every day.

The nutritional supplements and amounts listed above are those
supplements that work best for me.   You may consider using my
program as a starting point for your supplementation program.

There is more information on supplements, diet and exercise on
my Smartphone and Tablet APP, healthylc.

Dietary Guidelines

The diet part of the system provides guidelines to follow.   The guidelines will help you lower your stress response.

1. Minimize or eliminate sugar and wheat which acts like sugar from your diet.   Sugar is a concentrated carbohydrate that requires an abnormally high amount of water for its digestion.   It also enters the bloodstream rapidly.   The loss of body fluid coupled with the rapid increase in blood sugar raises the body's stress response and lowers energy levels.

2. Minimize or eliminate sodas from your diet.   Most sodas contain an acid that leaches the bones of calcium. Excess calcium in the blood stream thickens the blood, overworks the heart muscle, and increases the risk of arthritis.

3. Maintain your proper intake of protein.   For adults, it's 3 to 4 grams of protein per 10 pounds of weight.   Or, .3 to .4 times your weight in pounds.   You can go as high as 5 grams per 10 pounds of weight, but it depends on your age.   The higher amount of protein works if you are no more than 40 years old or are involved in heavy resistance training.

4. No concentrated proteins with your meals past 9 hours after waking up.   For most of us this is typically 5:00 PM.

This dietary practice will help to lower your stress response and promote the delivery of nutrients to the scalp which is necessary for hair growth.

5. Drink adequate amounts of water to stay hydrated.

MET Numbers for Various Levels of Activity

When comparing exercise routines, you can substitute routines that have the same MET number for the exercise routine you are engaged in.   In so doing, you avoid becoming bored with your routine.   Or, you can increase your daily level of activity by engaging in those that have a higher MET number.

MET of 3.0:

Stationary bike, light effort

Resistance training, light effort

MET of 3.5:

Cleaning house

Food shopping with a cart

Walking 3.0 mph

MET of 4.0:

Bicycle less than 10.0 mph

Shooting basketballs

Water aerobics

MET of 4.5:

Calisthenics

Dancing

Painting

MET of 5.0:

Stationary Bike, light effort

Aerobic dance, low impact

MET of 5.5:

Dance, fast

Mowing the lawn

MET of 6.0:

Bicycling 10 to 12 mph

Weight training, vigorous effort

Tennis, doubles

Bibliography

- American Publishing Corporation. Proven Health Tips Encyclopedia. Montclair:
- American Publishing Corporation, 1995.

- Atkins, Robert C.   Dr. Atkin's New Diet Revolution.   New York: HarperCollins Publishers, 2002.

- Brand-Miller, Jennie, and Kaye Foster-Powell, and Stephen Collaquiuri, and Thomas M. S. Wolever, and Anthony Leeds.   The Glucose Revolution.   New York: HarperCollins Publishers, 1999.

- Eades, Michael R., and Mary Dan Eades.   Protein Power.   New York: Bantam Books, 1999.

- Editors of Men's Health Magazine.   Men's Health Confidential. Emmaus: Rodale Press, 1988.

- Editors of Prevention Magazine.   Forever Young.   Emmaus: Rodale Press, 1988.
- Editors of Prevention Magazine.   Understanding Vitamins and Minerals.   Emmaus: Rodale Press, 1983.

- Greene, Bob, and Oprah Winfrey.   Make The Connection.   New York: Hyperion, 1996.

- Null, Gary.   Get Healthy Now.   New York: Seven Stories Press, 1999.

- Peters, Ken, and David Stuss, and Nick Waddell.   Hair Loss Prevention.   Vancouver: Apple Publishing Company, 1996.

- Pritikin, Nathan, and Patrick M. McGrady, Jr.   The Pritikin Program for Diet & Exercise.   New York: Bantam Books, 1979.

- Pritikin, Nathan.   The Pritikin Promise.   New York: Simon & Schuster, 1985.

- Sears, Barry, and William Lauren.   The Zone.   New York: HarperCollins Publishers, 1995.

- Whitney, Ellie, and Sharon Rady Rolfes.   Understanding Nutrition. Belmont: Thomson Wadsworth, 2005.

- www.pritikin.com. Updated date not provided.   Editors of the Pritikin Institute.   9 January 2008.